SomaVeda®
Integrated Traditional Therapies®

Thai Yoga
Breast Care Chirothesia Therapy
Certification Course

Second Edition

Anthony B. James
DNM, ND(T), MD(AM), DOM, PhD, RAAP

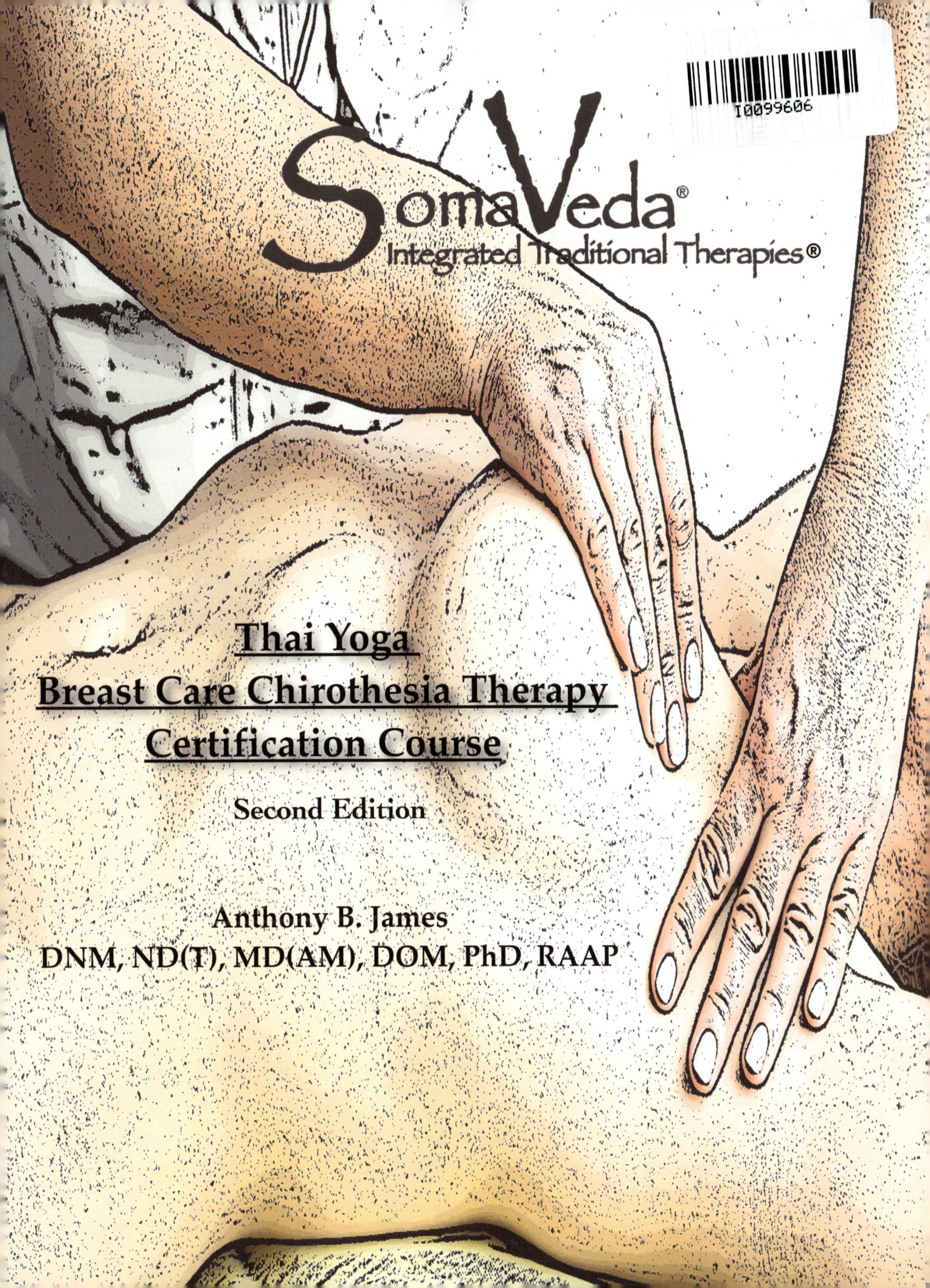

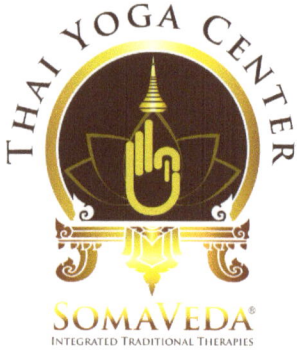

Native American Indigenous Church, Inc.
SomaVeda® Thai Yoga
Breast Care Chirothesia Therapy Certification
Workbook

Inquires should be addressed to:

Meta Journal Press

5401 Saving Grace Ln

Brooksville, Florida 34602

(706) 358-8687

e-mail NativeAIC@gmail.com

Web Site: www.ThaiYogaCenter.Com

ISBN-13: 978-1-886338-30-2

Breast Care & Therapy Certification

Purpose and description of the course:
SomaVeda® Breast Care & Therapy Certification Course (14 hours CE)

Breast health and care is as important as any other aspect of the spiritual, mental, emotional and physical health and wellbeing of our members. We believe that Breast focused therapeutics are vital and legitimate focus and work for healers when performed with informed consent and in an ethical, professional manner.

The Breast Care and Therapy certification program is intended to educate professional therapists in the major theories and information regarding natural and safe complementary preventative treatment protocols for breast health issues. SomaVeda® therapies offer possible benefits in reducing and or preventing risk factors and symptoms in breast related disorders; i.e. Breast Cancer, Fibromyalgia, Fibro Cystitis, Myalgias, Neuritis, Lymphedema, swelling, sensitivity and unwarranted soreness, Scar Tissue Contracture related to Breast Augmentation and Implants and Reconstructive Surgery, as well as "so called" breast related or "breast caused" back pain.

A ten step SomaVeda® protocol will be covered for implementing a professional, Therapeutic Breast Massage and Breast Care & Therapy Program. Hands on techniques of Decongestive Physiotherapy, Manual Lymph Drainage, Compression, Acupressure, Therapeutic Exercise, Skin Care and application of adjunct therapies will be covered in detail along with principles of risk reduction. Indications,
contraindications and possible side effects of the protocol will be covered, along with propriety, ethical and legal issues. The risk factors, issues of breast augmentation, circulatory factors of deficiency and toxemia, suppressed lymphatic activity and, brassiere related adverse heat and pressure will also be explored. The course includes anatomical and physiological focus of the relevant body region as well as self care breast massage for client's home use.

SomaVeda® Breast Care & Therapy and Healing programs are reserved for NAIC members only. A signed waiver/ informed consent will be required for participation.

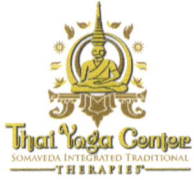

Pre-requisite: SomaVeda® practitioners/ counselors must be currently enrolled in a professional certification program and/or be currently NAIC Authorized Full Blessed Members (AFM) or equivalent: SMOCH, Priory of Saving Grace etc. ordained ministers. This course is in no way intended to represent medical advice or as a substitute for competent advice from a licensed medical professional. The opinions expressed herein are the opinion of the author, although supported by various sources and research, conclusions other than those expressed by the author may be drawn.

Why Breast Care and Therapy?

There is a major health crisis affecting women, their families, friends and businesses as well as the nation. Breast cancer is the number one critical health care issue today. It is the number one leading cause of death in women between the ages of 35 and 54. In 1960 the lifetime risk of having it was 1 in 20, today it is approaching 1 in 7. According to leading experts the number one risk factor for breast cancer is being a woman, 99% of all cases reported are in woman.

This year between 180,000 and 190,000 women will be diagnosed with breast cancer and approximately 44,000 will die from it. In addition to this consider the non cancerous or benign conditions, "Breast disorders", some of which are considered risk factors for these cancers. Our premise here is not that non-invasive and manual therapies can cure cancer, but rather they offer the benefits and assistance towards management of it, including pre and post-operative opportunities to reduce stress, pain, sensitivity, post op neurologic problems and edema. However, the research and experience do indicate that most if not all of the benign conditions can be moderated, if not reduced entirely, by Chirothesia based manual therapies.

Did you know that massaging your breasts is one of the most important routines of a woman's day? Our lymphatic system is responsible for keeping our body's tissues clean and healthy and for producing the cells that kill off bacteria, viruses and cancer cells in our body, i.e. our immune system. The lymphatic fluid that flows through our body to do this work is moved in three ways; respiration, muscle movement and manual manipulation. Without this movement, the fluid becomes stagnant and the tissue it permeates (fascia) becomes thicker and more uncomfortable, or diseased.

This fascial membrane is continuous throughout our bodies, and compression or congestion in one area affects the whole, causing aches, pains and swelling. Exercise is vitally important in moving this fluid. When we exercise, our muscles move, our breathing rate increases, and the lymph fluid is pumped around all body parts, except the breast!

The increase in flow to the breast is minimal as the breast tissue has no muscle. It lies atop the pectoral muscle in the chest. Add to that the fact that most women constantly restrict this area with a bra and it is easy to understand why breasts become painful and problematic.

External pressure and or manual manipulation is the only effective way to ensure fluid movement throughout the breast tissue. Manual Lymphatic Drainage focused emphasis, performed before, during and after breast massage, ensures that the lymph fluid from the breast has a pathway in which to drain.

Regular breast massage helps to keep tissue healthy and pain-free.

Benign Conditions

The benign conditions are not lethal, however, the concern that they may be precursors or risk factors in developing breast cancer, whether substantiated or not, causes much fear and trepidation making them extremely important to overall health and well being. They are generally described as the following: fibromyalgia, fibro cystitis, other myalgias, neuritis, lymphedema, generic swelling, sensitivity and unwarranted soreness, scar tissue contracture disorders, and so called "breast related back pain" or "breast caused back pain". We also want to include in the "issues" column more common conditions relating to Breast feeding and laction. The health and wellness of lactating mothers and those who want to naturally feed and support their children but who may have some difficulty doing so.

Preventing Unnecessary Surgury!

Every year hundreds of thousands of woman undergo expensive and risky treatments to address these benign conditions and with limited success. Annually thousands of women lose their breasts to mastectomy, perhaps unnecessarily, due to fear caused by these treatable conditions.

In general traditional western medicine does not offer much in the way of viable alternative, integrative and complementary protocols, instead choosing to rely on the convenience of drugs and surgery or worse. It is important to state here that we are not anti-conventional treatment when properly warranted. The author himself is a cancer survivor, who successfully underwent both surgical and chemical treatments to eradicate the disease. We believe however that the state of research into alternatives and especially in alternative therapies for benign conditions, is not accurately and fairly represented. In fact there is a growing body of evidence supporting that certain breast cancers may be avoidable, or cured by alternative means.

We feel that unfortunately most of the public information in the form of PSAs (Public Service Announcements) is skewed and politicized by special interest groups who seek to benefit from the diseases, especially the drug companies and their subsidiaries, the primary funders of basic research.

For example most basic research and public education relating to these matters is sponsored by the NCI (National Cancer Institute) and the ACS (American Cancer Society). These two along with a multitude of other not for profits, charities, runs, etc. all herald awareness through Breast Cancer Awareness Month. What most people do not know for example is that the primary sponsor and funding source of Breast Cancer Awareness Month is Zeneca Pharmaceuticals, now known as AstraZeneca. They own the patents and manufacture the widely distributed anti breast cancer drug Tamoxifin. They also are one of the largest producers of industrial pesticides, several of which are known to cause breast cancer! Several such Pharmaceutical companies have recently changed their names to avoid growing stigma and bad PR associated with growing public awareness of their roles in contributing to the growth of these and other types of Cancers.

There a possible conflict of interest here. We believe that carcinogenic substances, including pesticides are a major contributor to the "Causes" of breast cancer and related disorders, however, almost all of the public sector is narrowly focusing on the treatment of the symptoms. The left hand does not know what the right hand is doing. Yes, these ideas may be controversial, but if they spark debate and investigation then we are doing well. These mainstream sources would have us accept and believe that there are "No known avoidable causes of breast cancer". While at the same time promoting and distributing products proven to cause this and indeed many other different kinds of cancers. Tamoxifin for example is demonstrated in several studies to cause uterine cancer. This is referred to as a "substantial" side effect. I think it is more like trading one disorder for the possibility of another for profit at the expense of the public's welfare. Please do not take these comments out of context, refer to the sources and background material for support of any specific statistics and comments.

I am presenting this as an example of the social, economic, and political reasons that cause or contribute to all of the research and valid opinions not being fairly presented to the public. Vested interest in profit motives are dominant in ruling which theories and treatments are considered "legitimate". There seems to be especially significant resistance to any discussion of prevention or "avoidable risk factors". As these are the primary focus of Integrative and Complementary therapeutic approaches, virtually all such approaches are disparaged or ignored by the mainstream. However, a growing body politic is pushing for the whole story. There is growing acceptance of alternative therapies based on research being conducted around the world, studies which are outside the purview of NCI and ACS, which are not intended to generate patents for the production of income as their primary motive.

Thousands of years of Ayurveda, oriental and indigenous traditional medicine theory states clearly that true and effective cures address fundamental causes, more than symptoms.

This Breast and Chest Care wellness protocol addresses the Spiritual, Pycho-emotional, Physical and causative factors which all together manifest in Breast Disorder. This course is an attempt to step outside of the box and gain a more holistic and fair perspective on how manual procedures of SomaVeda® Complex Decongestive Therapy (SomaVeda® CDT) may help reduce some of the suffering in this growing community of Breast Cancer and Breast Disorder victims.

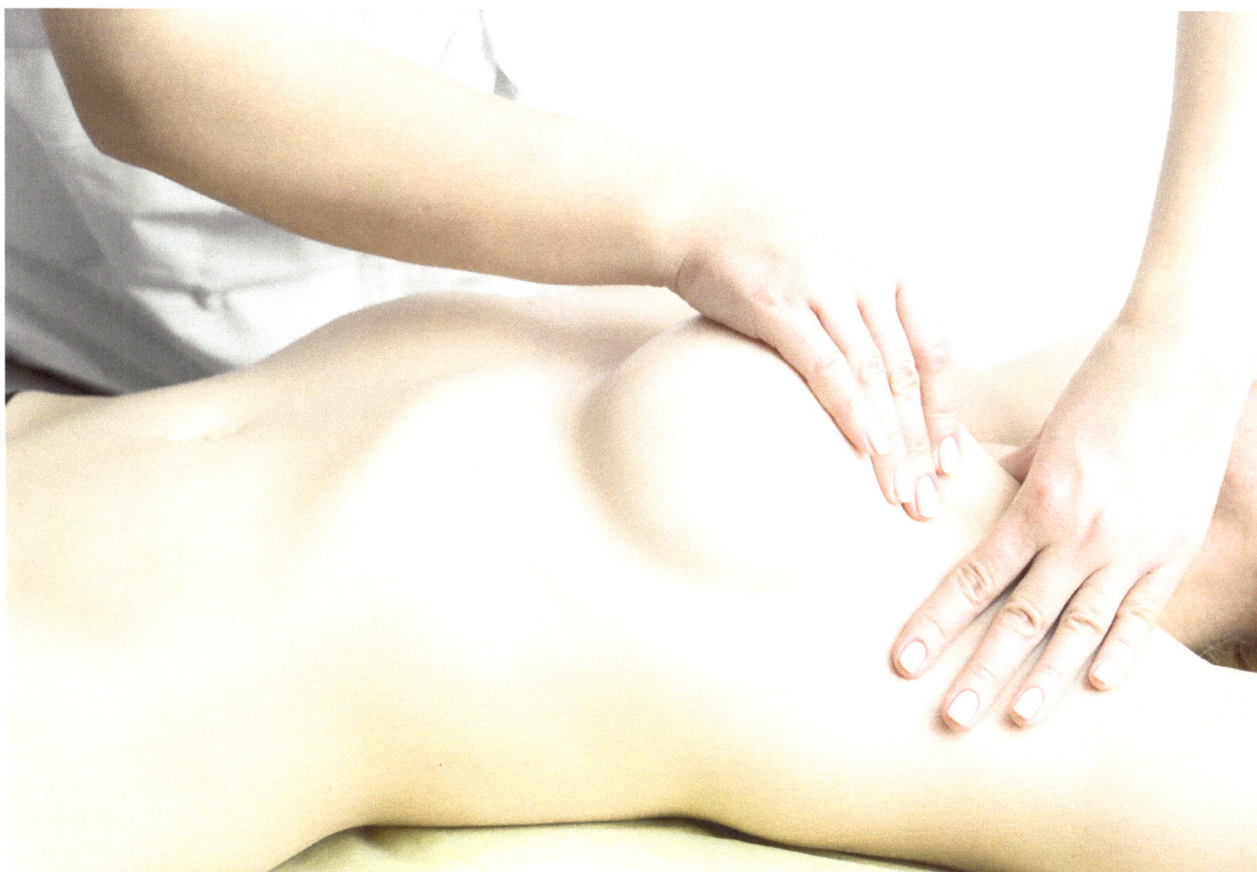

Ayurvedic Wisdom

Breast health is a vital component on the path to total wellbeing. Ayurveda, a 5,000-year-old healing wisdom tradition from India, teaches that in order to maintain a vibrant state of balance, the whole person must be addressed. In many healing practices the breasts are often overlooked as if including them was somehow inappropriate, but there are no bad body parts! Ayurvedic breast therapy addresses this gap in treatment to meet the needs of all women—healthy women, women who have been diagnosed with or are survivors of breast cancer, women who have fibrocystic breasts and women who are recovering from breast augmentation or reduction or cardiac abnormalities.

Chirothesia Massage is a way to nourish and maintain healthy breast tissue and musculature before potential issues arise, and to heal physically, emotionally and spiritually after life-changing disease such as breast cancer. Exercise is effective at pumping lymph fluid around every part of the body – except the breast. Yoga and Yoga Therapy with vibration and rocking are effective at pumping lymph fluid around every part of the body, except the breast, where the flow is often restricted by tight clothing. At the Thai Yoga Center we use the SomaVeda® Thai Yoga Chirothesia Breast Care Method (TYCBT) combined with traditional ayurvedic techniques and marma therapy for breast massage that helps to flush toxins through the lymphatic system, reduce pain, improve range of motion and increase the flow of prana (life energy).

The technique applies light strokes to mimic the pumping action of lymphatic vessels and encourages lymph flow. When healthy movement of the lymphatic fluid becomes restricted whether from compromised health, surgeries, restrictive clothing like bras, or even tense posture toxins can accumulate and lead to disease. The use of SomaVeda® CDT/ OPT protocols, TAELR™ instruments (tools) and adjuncts may be used as well, determined on an individual basis.

Utilizing the proprietary SomaVeda® Thai Yoga our Ayurvedic breast massage and Chirothesia Therapy helps to:

1) Flush toxins through the lymphatic system – Breast massage clears the lymphatic channels and ensures any toxins in the breast have a pathway to leave the body.

2) Reduce pain – When lymph fluid accumulates in one area, it affects the whole system, causing potential pain and swelling throughout the body. By opening up the lymph channels, Chirothesia breast massage helps to reduce pain not only in the breast, but the entire body.

3) Improve range of motion – Breast massage includes muscle release techniques to open up the shoulders and chest. In those who have had breast surgeries, this can restore range of motion that has been often severely restricted. This is also extremely beneficial for anyone who regularly sits at a desk, drives a car, or works at a computer.

4) Increase the flow of Prana/Breath – In Ayurveda, Prana is the vital energy that gives life to all beings. When the flow of Prana is restricted, we may experience symptoms such as fatigue, unhappiness, or illness. Breast massage provides the vital function of opening up the flow of Prana in the chest, gently removing energetic blocks around the heart that might otherwise remain unaddressed.

Our therapists perform the Ayurvedic breast massage, providing a healing touch (Chirothesia) that is customized specifically for the individual – taking into account their mind-body type (Dosha), medical history, and personal preferences. They provide a comfortable level of draping, and work with the client throughout the therapy so they can take part in their own healing.

Breast Cancer

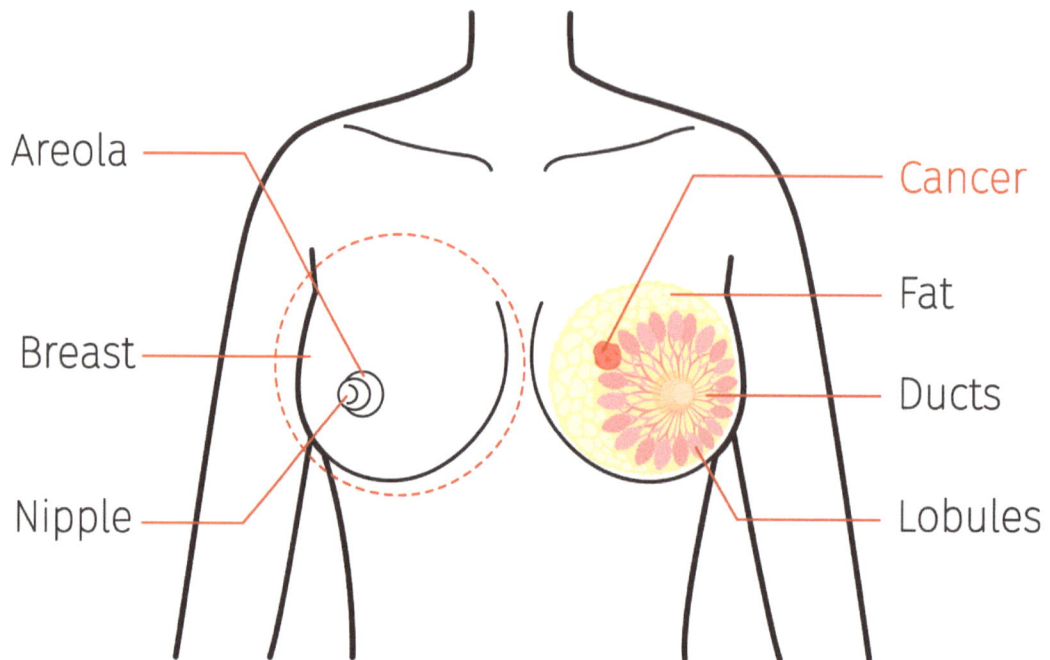

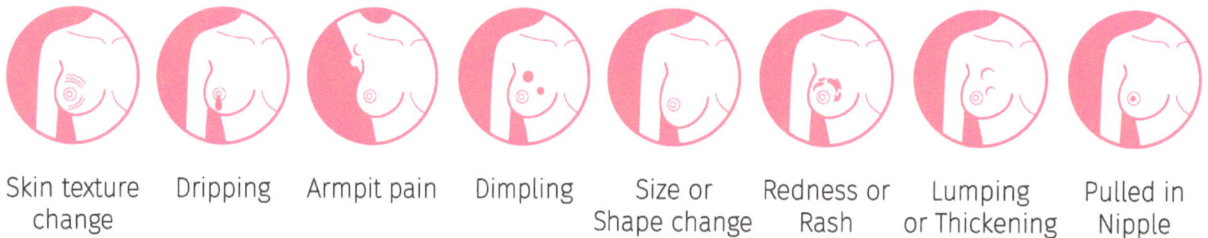

| Skin texture change | Dripping | Armpit pain | Dimpling | Size or Shape change | Redness or Rash | Lumping or Thickening | Pulled in Nipple |

Risk Factors for Breast Cancer

- •. Gender
- •. Increasing Age
- •. History of cancer in one breast
- •. History of benign breast disease or disorder
- •. Never giving birth or first pregnancy after age 30
- •. Family history (first degree relative) of breast cancer, (significant for premenopausal women)

- •. Early onset of menstruation and or late menopause
- •. History of cancer of the colon, thyroid, endometrium or ovary
- •. Chronic constipation
- •. Diet high in animal fat, excessive alcohol consumption and possible obesity
- •. Alterations in certain genes
- •. Breast implants
- •. Old Unresolved Negative Emotional Issues (NEMOs),(PTSD, Trauma)
- •. Spiritual Impairment: living out of synch with Spirit and Nature

We would add:

Long term wearing of bras as one if not the most important risk factor for breast cancer and breast disease or disorders.

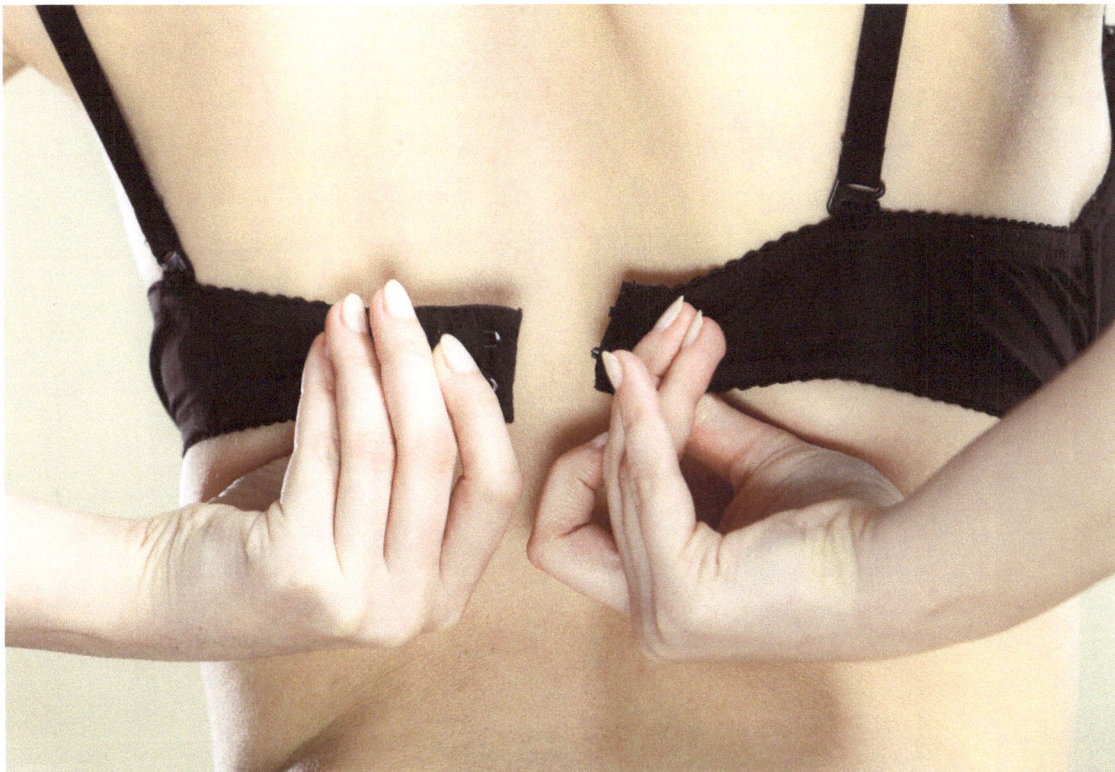

Consider a brassiere as more of a item of "costuming" that a necessity. Only use or wear when costuming! At the least only wear when socially orm professionally there is no other best option... At he least, reducing the time the breast are suspended in a "sling" position the more likely the suspensory ligaments will recover and the breast will naturally lift and assume a healthier look and feel. Typically this process takes 2 or more years to recover from a lifetime of wearing Bras!

Why might bras increase risk of cancer and breast disorder or disease?

They:

- •. Restrict blood flow
- •. Increase heat or local temperature
- •. Force shallow breathing
- •. Lower blood oxygen levels in the breast and surrounding area
- •. Increase breath rate
- •. Restrict lymphatic function
- •. Over stimulate key acupoints
- •. Contribute to fatigue
- •. Interfere with the free flow of energy, (i.e. Sen and Meridian)
- •. Cause lymphedema
- •. May contribute to reduction in melatonin levels in breast tissue
- •. Contribute to local increase of metabolic waste and toxins in breast tissue
- •. Impinge nerves causing stress and diminished function
- •. Impinge soft tissue, muscles and fascia causing trigger point syndromes
- •. May be a factor in chronic chest and back pain
- •. May contribute to development of cysts and fibrosclerotic tissue
- •. Increase risk of local infections
- •. Increase incidence of lympho cutaneous fistulas
- •. Increase incidence of fungal infections
- •. Decrease release of oxytocin to breast
- •. Cause or support scar tissue contracture disorder
- •. May contribute to difficulty, pain, discomfort in normal nursing or lactation.

Purposes of SomaVeda® TYCBT

1) Improvement of fatigue and quality of life.
2) Remove blockages and support the free flow of energy.
3) Increase blood flow within the breast and chest area, both arterial and venous.
4) Increase blood oxygen levels in the region.
5) Improve respiration quality.
6) Improve lymphatic function and circulation. (Lymphedema, left untreated may lead to invalidity or development of angiosarcoma - Stewart Treves Syndrome)
7) Normalize temperature.
8) Increase melatonin levels.
9) Reduce toxicity and residual metabolic wastes.
10) Increase available antioxidants.
11) Reduce accumulation of free radicals.
12) Normalize or reduce status of over stimulated pressure points.
13) Release or diminish scar tissue issues and contracture/ Decreased appearance of scars and stretch marks.
14) Reduce or eliminate edema and swelling
15) Reduce pain and sensitivity.
16) Reduce calcification and bone spurring caused by tight points of bras.
17) Improve or reduce effects of chronic venous insufficiency.
18) Reduce size and number of cysts.
19) Soften tissue by reducing fibrosclerotic tissue.
20) Reduce possibility of secondary infections.
21) Reduce Lymph Cysts.
22) Reduce lympho cutaneous fistulas.
23) Reduce varicose lymphatics.
24) Reduce fungal infections.
25) Stimulate release of oxytocin (increases blood flow).
26) Bring up, resolve, balance and address Spiritual, Pycho-emotional and energetic issues, Old Unresolved Negative Emotional Issues, trauma, and resolve, balance and or reduce their causative influence.
27) Decrease the symptoms of menstrual cramps.
28) Help with pain from surgery.
29) Reduce discomfort during pregnancy.
30) Improve your skin tone.
31) Increase breast milk production.
32) Provide relief from engorgement during breastfeeding.

33) Unblock plugged milk glands.
34) Can reduce stress and be deeply relaxing.
35) Toning of the muscles and connective tissue underlying, supporting breasts.
36) Natural breast enlargement and enhancement: In some women stimulates breast growth, resulting in a larger cup size. In others as it firms the tissue may reduce.
37) Reduce or eliminate tenderness or soreness in nipples.
38) Reduce bruising, wound (nipples areola, breast), fissures, ulceration, hemorrhages
39) Helpful in treating dermatitis: eczema, psoriasis (Use homeopathic application concurrent)

Additional Indications:

1) Pre/Post Surgical Interventions and Cosmetic Applications

2) Breast implant problems, post mastectomy, post lumpectomy, post tram flap, post lat flap, post breast reduction.

3) Improvement in local veno-lymphatic circulation, removal of toxins, tissue reoxygenation, regeneration of skin tissue, skin tonification, and mastoptosis (breast sagging), scars (acute and chronic)

The Human Breast

Anatomy & Physiology

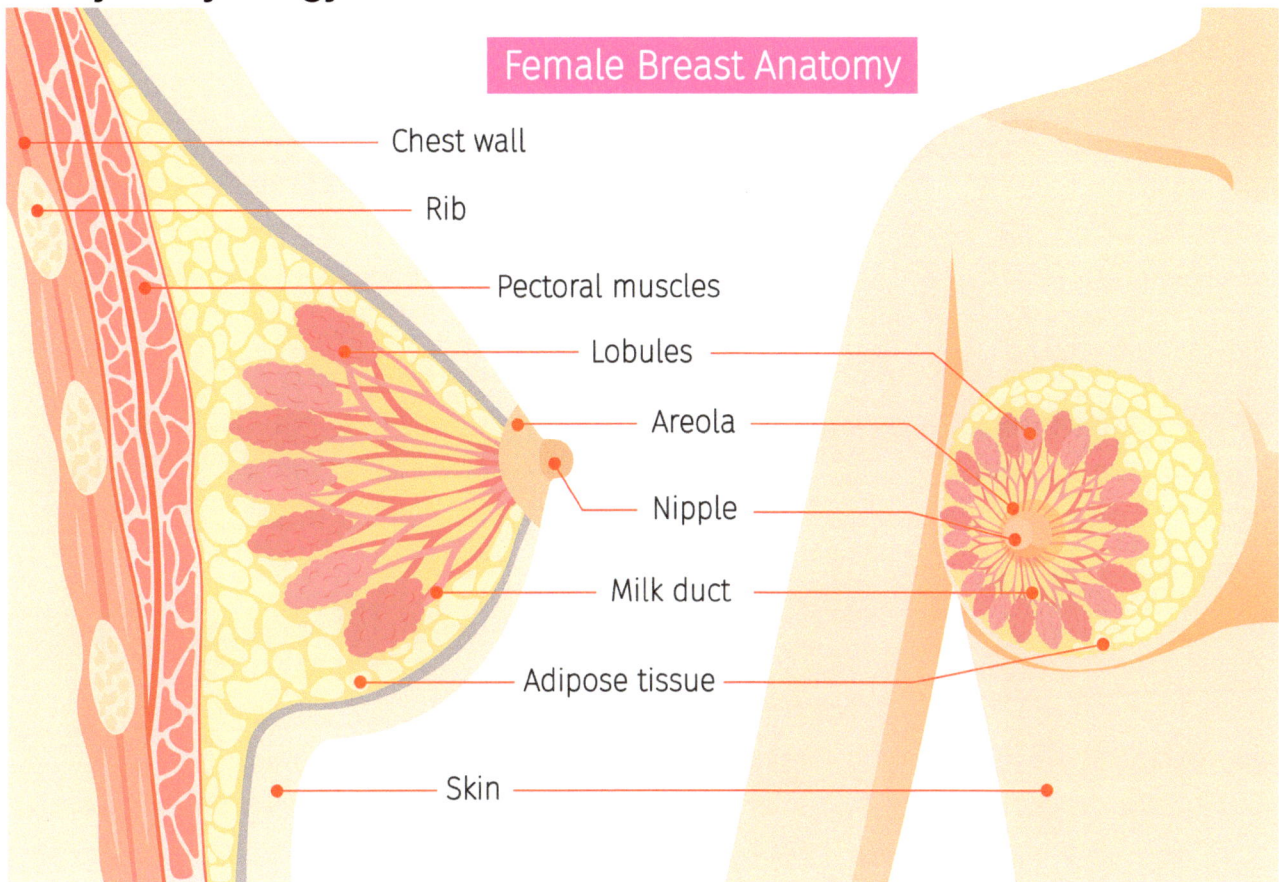

Female Breast Anatomy

- Chest wall
- Rib
- Pectoral muscles
- Lobules
- Areola
- Nipple
- Milk duct
- Adipose tissue
- Skin

The breast is a specialized gland structure that evolved essentially as an appendage of the skin. It develops within the layers of the subcutaneous superficial fascia. The most superficial of these fascial layers is positioned directly under the skin and forms the anterior boundary of the mammary gland. The deepest layer forms the posterior boundary and sits over the muscles of the chest wall. The tissues which make up the breast lie in between, anchored by extensions of these fascial membranes, and known as ligaments of Cooper or Cooper's Ligaments. These thickened fascial strands extend into the breast to provide a supporting framework. Cooper's Ligaments are also called the suspensory ligaments.

Deep to the point where the breast attaches to the posterior layer of the superficial fascia is a zone of loose areolar tissue called the retromammary space. The arrangement of looseconnective tissue in this space allows the breast to move fairly freely over the fascia covering pectoralis major. The retromammary space also plays an important role in the lymphatic drainage of the breast, as we will discuss shortly.

The rounded contour of the breast projects anteriorly from the chest wall and suspends loosely against gravity. There are no muscles or cartilaginous structures within the breast, so it relies on its fascial envelope and suspensory ligaments for integrity and support. This information is important for the massage therapist, who should avoid techniques that could unduly stress or stretch these structures.

In the center of the breast's surface is a circle of darker skin called the areola. While usually a somewhat deeper version of the woman's skin color, the areola can become very dark in high estrogen states like pregnancy. The skin of the areola contains a large number of specialized sebaceous glands, referred to as Montgomery's glands, which are clearly visible as small bumps.

The nipple is positioned at the centre of the areola. Both the subareolar tissue and the nipple are richly supplied with smooth muscle that runs in both circular and radiating patterns. When these muscle fibers contract the nipple erects, and if the woman is lactating, the milk sinuses empty. The nipple is also a centre of sexual sensation and is served by a large number of sensory nerve endings.

Breast tissue extends beyond the breast contour. Look closely and compare the protuberant breast contours (left breast) with the boundaries of mammary tissue as shown on the right side. This information about the actual extent of breast tissue is very important to the practitioner because findings of breast tissue tenderness, nodularity, and benign and malignant lumps may all occur in this larger zone beyond the contours of the breast. These thin, extended layers may also swell painfully with inflamed or engorged breasts.

The breast overlies several muscles. On average, 50% of the breast sits over pectoralis major, and the rest over the other muscles of the chest wall, especially serratus anterior. Variable small amounts of breast tissue overlie latissimus dorsi superolaterally, and the lower edge covers a bit of rectus abdominis.

It is common and quite normal for a woman's breasts to be two different sizes. The most common breast abnormality is presence of one or more accessory nipples, usually found along the "nipple line" in the abdomen. Another frequently occurring breast irregularity is a greater than average extension of breast tissue into the axilla. It is important to be aware of this anomaly, because it can look like a mass. The tissue will not appear ominous in that it is malleable, its boundaries are soft and easily palpated, and it moves well in relation to nearby tissue. Medical examination is necessary, however, to ensure the formation is simply extra breast tissue.

The breast is made of lobes of glandular tissue with associated ducts for transfer of the milk to the exterior and supportive fibrous and fatty tissue. About 80-85% of normal breast tissue is fat during the reproductive years. The 15-25 lobes are further divided into lobules containing alveoli (small sac like features) of secretory cells with smaller ducts that conduct the milk to larger ducts and finally to a reservoir that lies just under the nipple. In the nonpregnant, nonlactating breast, the alveoli are small. During pregnancy, the alveoli enlarge and during lactation the cells secrete milk substances, i.e. proteins and lipids. Muscular cells surrounding the alveoli contract to express the milk during lactation. Breast tissue is supported by ligaments called Cooper's ligaments that keep the breasts in their characteristic shape and position. In the elderly or in pregnancy these ligaments become loose or stretched, respectively, and the breasts sag.

Reproductive hormones are important in the development of the breast in puberty and in lactation. Estrogen promotes the growth of the gland and ducts while progesterone stimulates the development of milk producing cells. Prolactin, released from the anterior pituitary gland, stimulates milk production. Oxytocin, released from the posterior pituitary in response to suckling, causes milk ejection from the lactating breast.

The lymphatic system drains the tissues of the breast of excess fluid. Lymph nodes along the pathway of drainage screen for foreign bodies such as bacteria or viruses. The lymph nodes can also become enlarged when migrating cancer cells get lodged in the nodes. This is why lymph nodes located in the armpit are checked during a breast exam and why they are often cut out along with cancerous tissue in the treatment of breast cancer.

Puberty and Maturity

In response to hormone stimulation, the breasts enlarge due to the growth of ductal and alveolar tissues and an increase in fat deposits. The nipple and areola also enlarge and become more sensitive to touch. When the woman begins to menstruate, the breasts undergo a periodic premenstrual phase that varies with the individual but can include an increase in size, swelling and tenderness. The symptoms subside within a few days of the onset of bleeding. During pregnancy, the breasts increase in size dramatically due to the influence of progesterone. The nipple and areola become deeply pigmented and increase in size. Most of the fat is replaced by the necessary machinery to produce milk by late pregnancy. After delivery the breasts begin to secrete milk. The gland rapidly returns to the prepregnant state when nursing ceases. The postmenopausal breast may retain its shape but the milk producing machinery is mostly replaced by fat.

Lactation

The breasts become fully developed under the influence of estrogen, progesterone and prolactin during pregnancy. Prolactin causes the production of milk, and oxytocin release (via the suckling reflex) causes the contraction of smooth muscle cells in the ducts to eject the milk from the nipple. The first secretion of the mammary gland after delivery is called colostrum. It contains more protein and less fat than subsequent milk and contains antibodies that impart some passive immunity to the infant. Most of the time it takes 1-3 days after delivery for milk production to reach appreciable levels. The drop in circulating estrogen and progesterone caused by the expulsion of the placenta at delivery initiates milk production. Estrogen antagonizes the positive effect of prolactin on milk production. The physical stimulation of suckling causes the release of oxytocin and stimulates prolactin secretion stimulating more milk production.

Successful Breastfeeding Poster

Benefits to the Breastfed Infant

It lessens the risk of being an obese later in life

Protects your baby from infections and diseases

Less chance of developing eczema

Less chance of diarrhoea and vomiting

They are less likely to die of SIDS

Natural food designed for your baby

They have fewer ear infections

It makes nappies less smelly

They have better vision

They have better skin

They have healthier brains IQ

decreased anxiety

increased confidence

It can give you a great sense of achievement

Whats'In Breast Milk?
Breast milk is a unique combination of nutrients essential to a child's health

1% proteins
87% water 7% carbohydrates
vitamins fats
minerals 1%
hormones 1% 4%

Breastfeeding results in less sick days for parents

Breastfeeding satisfies baby's emotional needs

Better social development

Breast milk provides superior nutrition and immunoprotection to the infant. Indeed, infants breastfed for six months have a lower risk of respiratory infections in the first two years as compared to infants breastfed for only four months. Breastfeeding also decreases the risk of recurrent ear infections and is protective against gastrointestinal infections.

Benign Breast Tumors

These include fibroadenoma, periductal fibromas (connective tissue tumor), intraductal epithelial tumor, retention cysts, lipomas (fatty tumor), chronic cystic mastitis and fat necrosis. Most often they occur during the reproductive period of life or just after. These are often difficult to distinguish from malignant tumors and must be watched for a change in size, or lymphatic involvement, in which case the growth should be cut out and examined. Mammograms, ultrasound, thermography and aspiration of cystic forms can aid in diagnosis. Most non-malignant masses in the breast will resolve or diminish quickly with regular Breast Care.

Fibrocystic Breast Disease

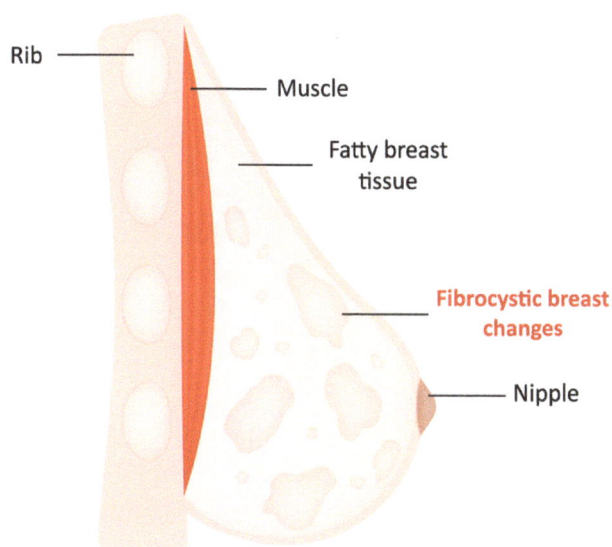

Healthy Breast

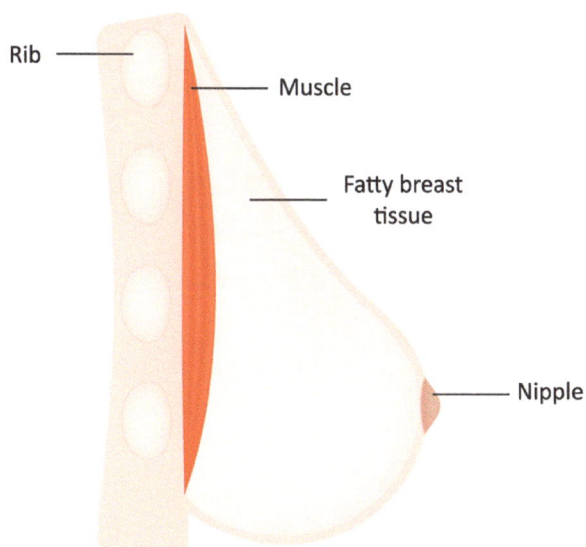

Rib ———

——— Muscle

——— Fatty breast tissue

——— Nipple

Fibrocystic Breast Disease

Rib ———

——— Muscle

——— Fatty breast tissue

——— **Fibrocystic breast changes**

——— Nipple

Malignant Breast Tumors

Breast cancer is the most common type of cancer in women and is a major public health problem in the U.S. with 1 in 8 women expected to be diagnosed sometime during their lives. Cancers of the breast are treated by several measures dependent on the patient's age, clinical status, the type and size of the tumor, the degree of spread, and the estrogen responsiveness of the tumor. Some 35% of cancer of the breast in women of childbearing age are estrogen-dependent, meaning that their continued growth is dependent on the presence of estrogen. Symptoms are often dramatically decreased by the removal of the ovaries, the major source of estrogen. Breast cancer in males occurs but is rare.

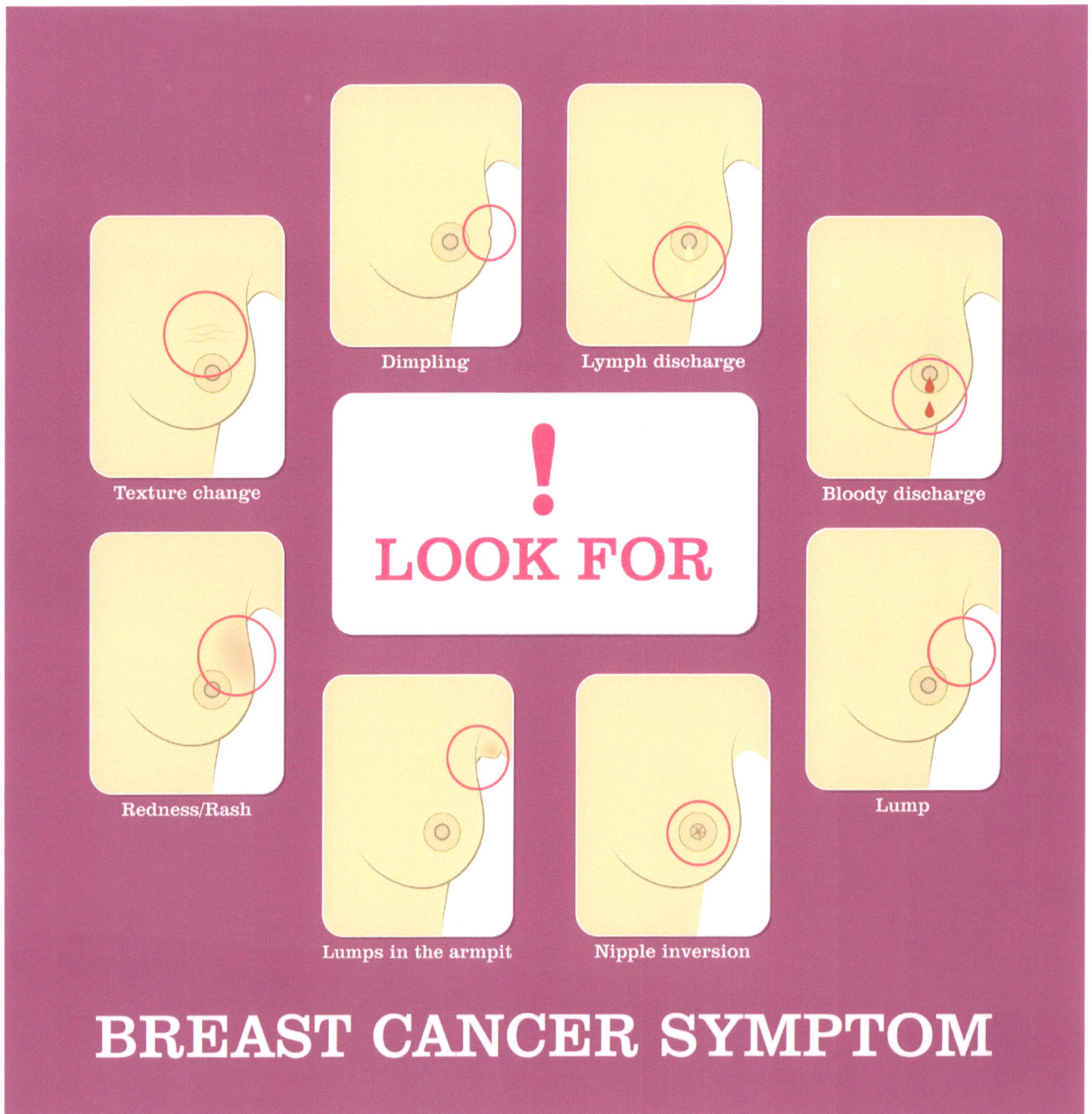

Texture change

Dimpling

Lymph discharge

Bloody discharge

! LOOK FOR

Redness/Rash

Lumps in the armpit

Nipple inversion

Lump

BREAST CANCER SYMPTOM

Risk factors associated with breast cancer are:

*   beginning menstruation early &/or late menopause.
*   no children or children born after age 30.
*   history of fibrocystic disease.
*   family history of breast cancer.

Signs Suggestive of Breast Cancer (1) (Seek Physician's advice):

1) Painless lumps (only 5-7% of cancerous lumps are painful)
2) Hard lumps fixed to the surrounding tissue, rapidly increasing in size, no change to hormonal cycles
3) Alterations in the skin. Orange-peel appearance, eczema of the nipple, unexplained lesions, unexplained skin breakdown, skin ulceration
4) Changes in breast contour, breast thickening
5) Nipple discharge, especially bloody or dark brown (about 5% of these are malignant in origin)
6) Nipple retraction
7) Inflammatory signs- redness of the skin, pain, swelling
8) Breast varicosities- enlarged superficial veins

Breast cancer is usually detected by self exam where the woman finds a lump that is painless, non tender and movable. In more advanced cases the lump becomes anchored to the underlying muscle. The skin may show signs of the cancer by dimpling or retraction. Mammography, thermography, and ultrasound may be used for diagnosis. Breast biopsy is used for confirmation of diagnosis. Treatment can include surgery in the form of lumpectomy or mastectomy, sometimes followed by radiation, chemotherapy or endocrine therapy unless CAM Therapy is indicated.

Breast Self Exam

Many medical personnel can provide instruction for performing a breast self exam. This procedure should be done monthly shortly after the menstrual period because the changes induced in the breast by progesterone may confuse results. The procedure should also be done monthly after menopause. If any abnormality is discovered, a physician should be contacted.

A physician will generally palpate the breasts in a similar manner during a physical exam. The basic steps include:

*   Lie down with one hand behind your head.
*   With the other hand, gently feel the extended breast, pressing lightly, with flattened fingers. Begin at the outer axillary portion (near arm pit) and move in a circular clockwise pattern inwardly toward the nipple. Gently feel for lumps or thickening's. Remember to feel all parts of the breast, including the underarm area.
*   Repeat the same procedure sitting up with the hand still behind your head.
*   Repeat the above steps for the other breast.

Gynecomastia

This is breast development in the male caused by a shift in the estrogen:androgen ratio due to increased circulating estrogen or a decrease in circulating androgens. But there may be multiple causes. For instance, digoxin can cause gynecomastia infrequently because it is weakly estrogenic. The diuretic spironolactone can also cause gynecomastia.

General principles in preparation and administration.

Have client fill out and sign an informed consent form.

Create and maintain a safe, clean environment, free of unwarranted interruption.

If indications of cancer are present, do not perform therapy on any possibly cancerous area without a specific physicians consent.

Hands and fingernails must be clean.

Keep client warm and comfortable.

Use draping where appropriate and only un-drape actual area necessary to be worked on and with consent of client. Always ask before exposing the breast directly, even if it was discussed at the beginning of the session. Think, "That was then, this is now".

No hard or pointed pressure on the breast as you want to avoid any bruising.

10 Step Protocol
(SomaVeda® Thai Yoga Chirothesia Breast Care Method (TYCBT))

#1 Warm up:
   a) Work Points, Wind Gates (lom) in shoulder/ arm area. (PP, TP)
   b) Work Neck Points and lines with light compression (Palm, Rolling Thumb)
   c) Axilla and Breast Pull and Push 3 angles with Hooking Fingers and Compression
   d) Abdominal massage (Level 2 or 3 protocol)

#2 Circles: Finger Circles, sternum to clavicle 3X, Palm circle entire torso in figure 8 pattern, 3X
   "Level Three"style

#3 Pressure Points: TP pressure points between ribs (Level Three Style)

#4 Circles Again: a) Finger Circles around perimeter of breast 3X.
   b) Finger circles, cover entire breast in a spiral pattern from outside to inside.

#5 V-Hand bilateral compression: 3 positions (3 different angles).

#6 Torque/ Rotate: Gentle twist with compression (whole hand), press inward, 3X.
   Twist both directions.

#7 Draw The Lines: 8 Lines. Finger drag inside to out, in a radial fashion.

#8 Palm circles: with thumb lock on the nipple (Do not pinch)

#9 Squeeze/ Compression: Gently squeeze and twist the nipple area including aureole. (Stimulates release of Oxytocin, increasing blood flow)

#10 Vibration: Gently shake and or jostle. (Shensen= vibration)

Optional Steps / Adjuncts

1) SomaVeda® T.A.E.L.R.™: (Tool Assisted Energy Line Release & Gua Sha) with hand tool all lines and surfaces of the Arms, Axilla, Chest and Breast.

2) Vibratory Endermatherapy: using electro-mechanical device (PureWave or other Professional Mechanical Vibrator). Same procedure as for Thai "Gua Sha" using device.

3) Photobiomodulation/ Light Therapy: using Far-Infrared light device. 15 to 45 min depending on power of device.

4) CDT Protocol: using High-frequency device and appropriate wands. May also use iodine application with high frequency iontophoresis. Paint iodine over breast surface - then use wand. Discoloration will go away shortly as iodine (Lugol's) is absorbed.

5) SomaVeda® Nuad Prakhop Samun Praii (Steamed Herbal Poultice)

6) SomaVeda® BET for emotional issues relating to the breast and or any related issues that surface during protocol.

7) Sacred Nutritional Counseling: addressing eating habits, plant based diet and supplemental food strategies... i.e. Fulvic Minerals, Sacred Waters-Iodine, Sacro-Flora Pro10 Probiotics, Balanced meal replacement product, Juicing etc. Anti-inflamatory Ayurvedic nutritional suppliments (Curcumen, Tumeric etc.)

8) Self treatment: coaching and instruction.

9) SomaVeda® Therapeutic Day Protocol!

10) Suitable Yoga program.

11) Advanced Only! As part of initial assessment perform the the visual and Breast Temperature/ Thermographic survey using Infrared Thermometer or FLIR camera. Use proper form and note all temps and mean variation numbers. If outside accepted variation refer for medical thermography clinical assessment.

Sample Session with Detox Protocol

1) Intake procedure: A full and complete medical and or clinical assessment is indicated. If qualified as a St. John POC technician/ technologist then all clinical assessments are useful.

If a standalone session then the BET/ EFT must be implemented as well. It is appropriate for NAIC Minister/ Practitioners to also suggest and or conduct Chirothesia/ and or ceremony such as Sweat, Pipe, Breath Blessing, Tobacco, Smudging etc. as complementary therapies.

2) Puja and Warm up the tissue: Prepare client by wrapping warm / steamed towels over the breast area for 3 to 5 min.

3) Anointing: Use a light oil or lotion to do Basic 10 Step Protocol. (May be done dry)

4) Purification: Light exfoliation with, towel, brush or mitt. May also use a natural product such as an apricot scrub. If a granular product is used, it must be washed and removed.

5) Wash: Light body shampoo of the area, with rinse and towel wipe.

6) Cleanse Toxins: Apply a good cleansing and or detox mask. May use herbal, mineral (mud) or veggie type. Wait prescribed time and remove. Clean up residue.

7) Oliation/ Annointing: Use oil for light decongestive, lymphatic Chirothesia massage. Use Aromatherapy oils if desired. Any good quality, non-GMO, non- toxic oil including Ghee is useable.

8) Sweat: Apply Steam towels or steamed herbal compress. (A healing sweat by natural means, far infrared sauna, Ozone/ Oxygen, are also perfect adjuncts.)

9) Clean Up: Dry and allow 3 to 5 min meditation, rest.

10) PranaYama & Puja: complete with 3 to 5 min. Breath, Pranayama, Prayer and or Puja.

Additional Breast Health, Care and Public Interest Articles and resources

Lymph

In addition to the blood vascular system, the body contains a network of thin walled vessels that act to remove excess extracellular fluid from the tissues and return it to the blood. Fluid leaves the vascular system across capillary walls at a greater rate than it returns, such that another system is necessary to return excess fluid to the blood system. Lymph is composed of water, ions, protein, clotting factors, lymphocytes, and fats absorbed from the intestine. Lymph collected from the tissues is transported along thin-walled valved vessels to larger lymph vessels to drain into the venous blood via the thoracic and right lymphatic ducts. Large lymphatics have poorly developed tunics and many more valves than veins.

Lymphatic Circulation and The Breast

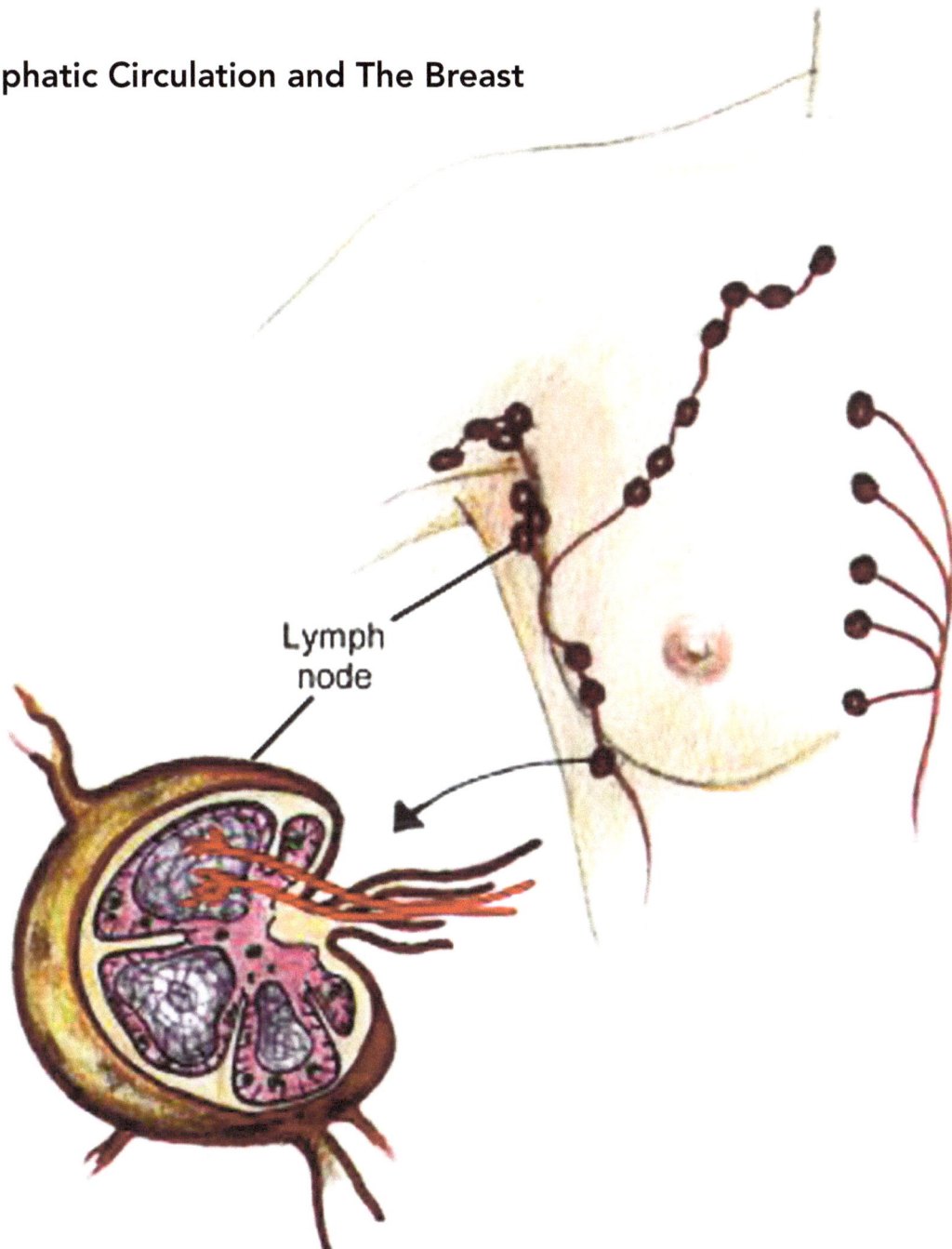

Lymph
node

These thin walled channels are lined with endothelium and in the case of the larger vessels are similar in structure to veins with limited adventitial development. The channels begin in the tissue as very thin closed end vessels. Lymphatic capillaries are more porous than vascular capillaries because they lack tight junctions between endothelial cells and have a very limited basal lamina. Lymphatics are found in most all organ systems with the notable exceptions of the central nervous system and bone marrow.

Lymph is moved along within the system mostly by the action of external forces such as muscle contractions or changes in intrathoracic pressure with respiration. However, distention of the larger lymph vessels causes contractions of the ducts that propel the lymph along.

The lymphatic system contains nodes that act as in-line filters to remove antigens and debris from

Pattern of drainage for Lymphatic network, nodes and capillary.

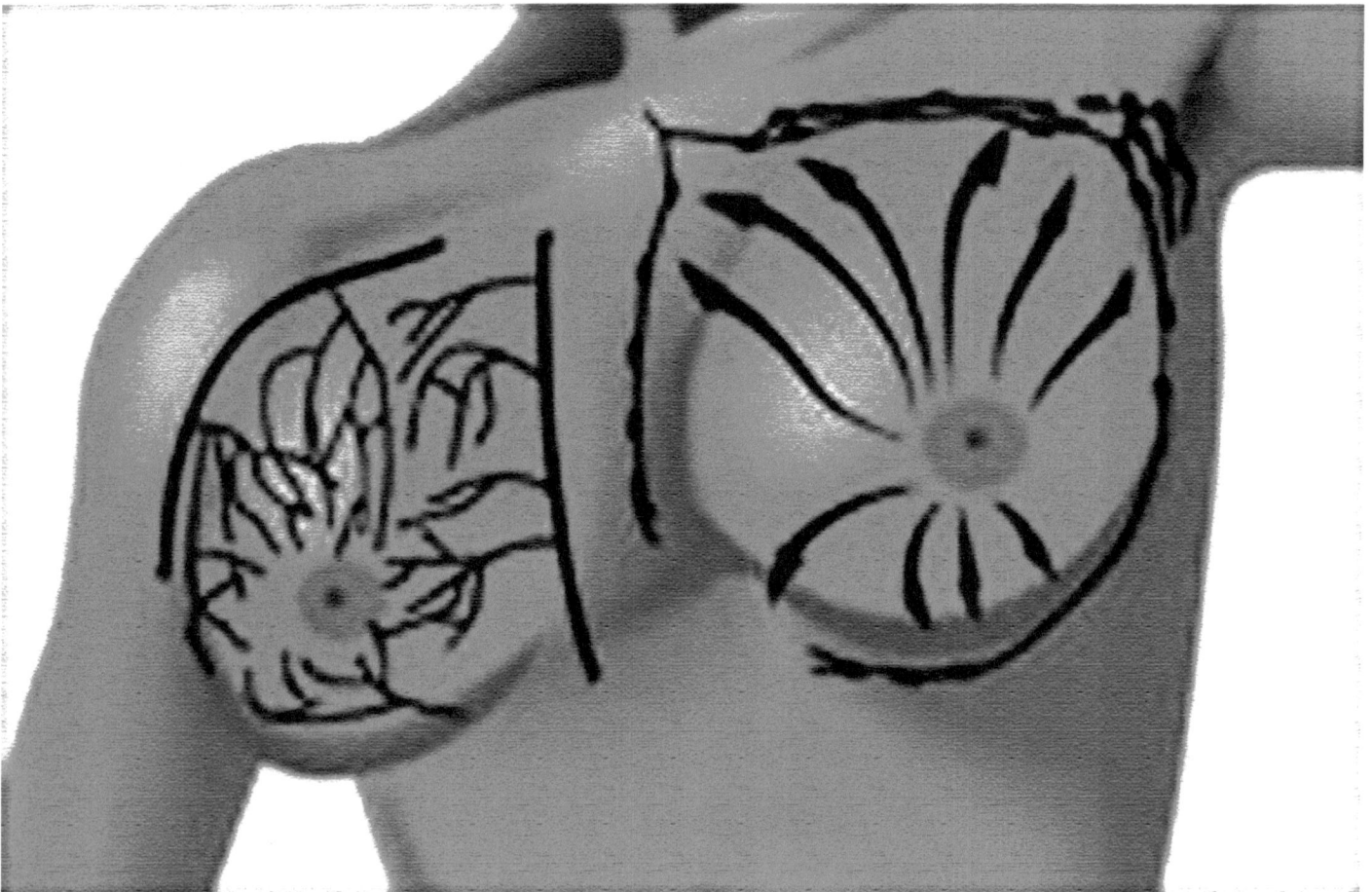

the lymph prior to its return to the blood. The node are spherical or kidney shaped structures found in the axilla, groin, neck, thorax and abdomen. The distribution of these nodes is such that all collected tissue fluid is filtered at least once before returning to the bloodstream. Macrophages lodged in the nodes remove microorganisms and debris by phagocytosis and the numerous lymphocytes housed there have first exposure to infectious agents so as to mount a humoral defense. Malignant tumor cells are often caught and spread from peripheral satellite nodes.

The lymphatic system returns proteins from the interstitial fluid of the liver and intestine to the blood vascular system, helps to maintain the renal concentrating ability, and transports in lipoproteins, fats, long-chain fatty acids and cholesterol absorbed in the intestine. The lymphatics are necessary for the maintenance of normal tissue fluid levels.

Edema

Obstruction of the lymphatics can cause regional accumulation of fluid known as edema. Edema is harmful because the delivery of nutrients and removal of wastes is impeded by increased tissue fluid pressures and diffusion distances. Gravity contributes to edema in dependent parts as does the retention of salt in the body. Certain parasites have a preference for the lymphatics and can cause edema via the obstruction of the lymph capillaries. Another cause of obstruction is metastatic infiltration and obstruction of the lymph nodes and vessels. Malnutrition can cause edema as well due to a decrease in plasma oncotic pressure (decreased plasma proteins) which would normally oppose movement of water into the tissues. High blood pressures or increases in capillary permeability also can precipitate edema.

The causes of edema are classified as lymphangitis when the lymph vessels are inflamed due to bacterial infection most commonly by streptococci, lymphadenitis when lymph nodes are inflamed, and lymphedema when the edema results from obstruction. Source Altrus Biomedical Network: © Altruis LLC 2002, http://www.e-breasts.net

Regular breast massage helps to keep tissue healthy and pain-free.

SUGGESTED Workshop Format:

TITLE: The Art of SomaVeda® Thai Yoga Chirothesia Breast Care Therapy in Supporting Lactation and Breastfeeding Workshop

Overview:

Breast pain is one of the major causes of weaning. The likelihood of weaning increases the longer pain persists. Engorgement, plugged ducts, blebs and mastitis are commonly associated with acute breast pain. Therapeutic Thai Yoga Breast Therapy in Lactation (TYCBT) is one of the important measures to resolve pain quickly.

The purpose of this workshop is to enhance knowledge of TYCBT techniques for relieving discomfort caused by engorgement, plugged ducts and mastitis in lactating women and learn how to empower breastfeeding mothers to use these techniques as well.

Objectives:

1) Describe how breast Care and Therapy is used by different cultures to help with problems such as engorgement, plugged ducts, and mastitis.
2) Identify causes of acute breast pain and treatment options.
3) Describe how hand expression and therapeutic breast therapy (TYCBT) assist in management of engorgement, plugged ducts and mastitis.
4) Demonstrate and teach lactation consultants simple techniques of SomaVeda® breast massage and hand expression.
5) Explain how to teach self-breast care and therapy techniques to breastfeeding mothers

Schedule:

8:30-9:00 - Registrations and Welcome

9:00-10:15 - Breast Therapy and Hand Expression

10:15-10:30 - Break

10:30-11:45 - Using the Hands to deal with the Pain: Therapeutic Breast Therapy in Lactation: research and case reviews

11:45-12:00 - Break

12:00 -1:15 Lunch Break

1:15-2:45 - Hands on Practice Group

2:45-3:00 - Break

3:00- 4:30 - Teaching TYBT Techniques, Self-breast Massage and Hand Expression

4:30-5:00 - Discussion, Q&A and Evaluation

NAIC/ Somaveda College of Natural Medicine: CE's will be provided.

www.ingramcontent.com/pod-product-compliance
Lightning Source LLC
Chambersburg PA
CBHW060900270326
41935CB00003B/45